HOPE

April 2018

After Brain Injury

HOPE
MAGAZINE

"Supporting the
Brain Injury Community"

HOPE MAGAZINE

Serving All Impacted by Brain Injury

April 2018

Publisher
David A. Grant

Editor
Sarah Grant

Contributing Writers
Ali Blaylock
Virginia Cote
Debra Gorman
Jim Martin
Mark Moore
Ted Stachulski
Michelle Stokes
Seth Williams

*FREE subscriptions at
www.HopeAfterBrainInjury.com*

Welcome to the April 2018 issue of HOPE Magazine!

A recent comment on Facebook caught my attention and brought a smile to my face. When a reference was made to HOPE Magazine, the reply was just wonderful.

"I love that magazine!'

Over the last several years, we have quietly and steadily made inroads to the brain injury community worldwide. From individual readers in over forty countries to statewide brain injury associations and area agencies, every month, our publication lands in the hands of those who need it most.

I am no newbie to brain injury. Now in year eight as a survivor, I often wonder what it would have been like if my wife Sarah and I had a resource like HOPE Magazine to turn to.

We would have known that we weren't alone and that there were others who shared our fate.

This month's issue has remarkable stories of courage and survival. If you've become a regular reader, welcome back. If you are a new reader, welcome. You will find hope here.

Peace,

David A. Grant
Publisher

Contents

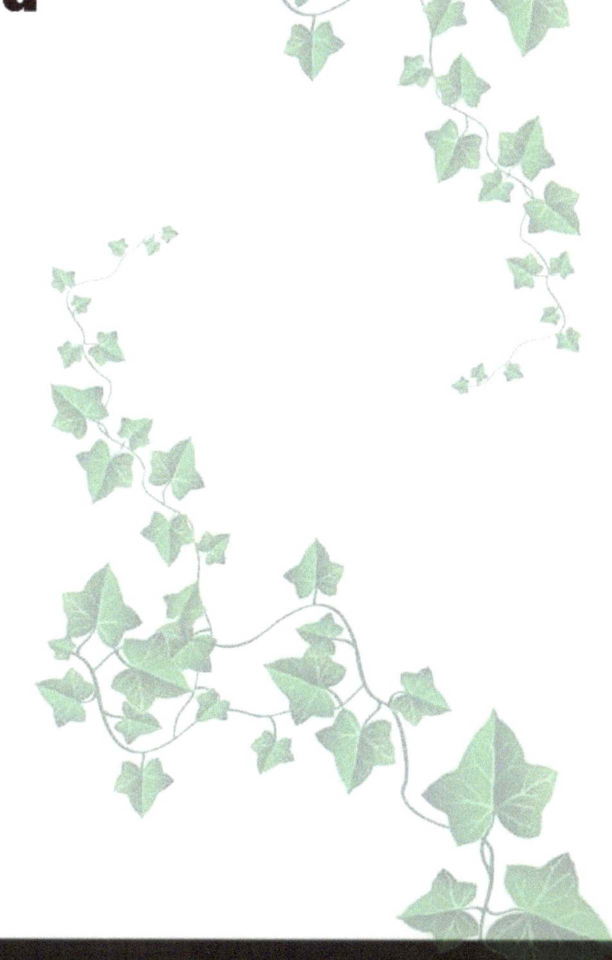

"Few things in the world are more powerful than a positive push."

~Richard DeVos

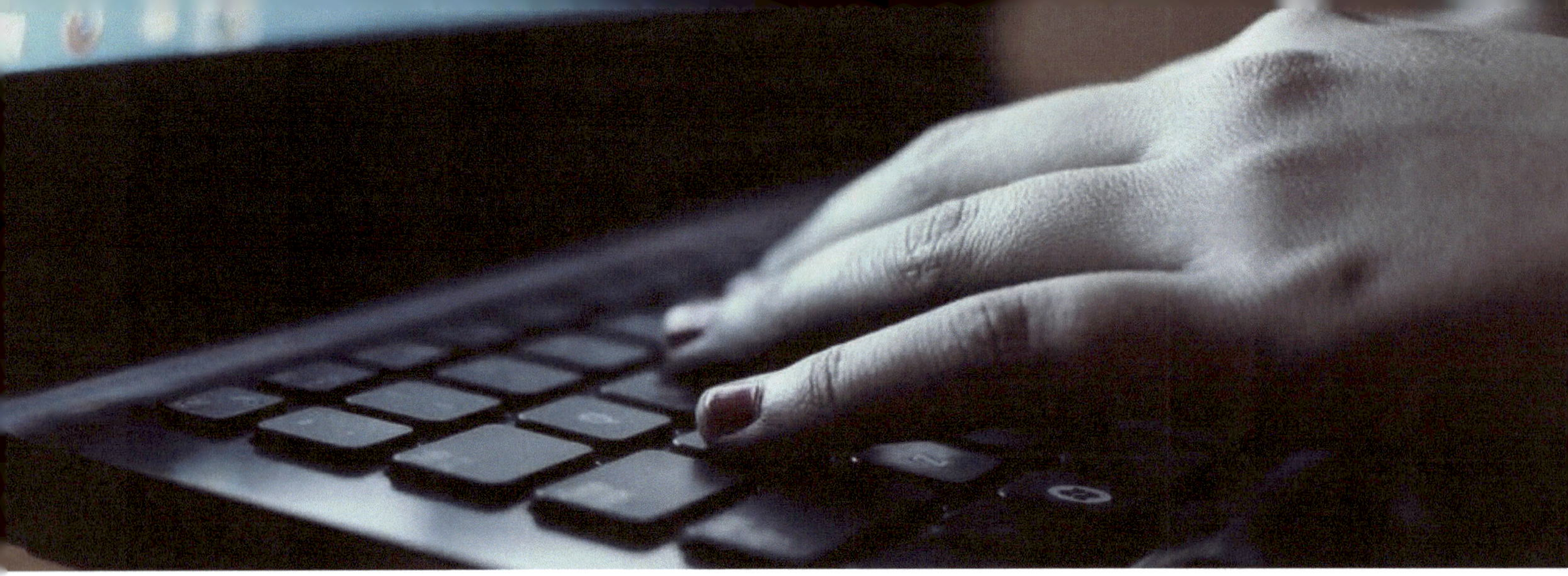

Brain Injury Glitches
By Ali Blaylock

Just imagine that you have a top-of-the line computer capable of processing complex information, linking to multiple sources of existing and new data, and formulating innovative and fresh ideas. One day its cord gets tugged and a plug comes undone. It looks fine, but after it is hooked back up, there are some "mild glitches," according to the troubleshooter.

Computers are expensive and it is only a "mild" problem, so you optimistically take it to one of the best computer repair shops for evaluation.

They diagnose malfunctions in the wiring and hard drive that corrupt, misfile and delete stored data, turn organized informational pathways into spaghetti, and randomly apply distortion filters to images or audio. Input from external sources is frequently garbled, misdirected, and misinterpreted. Part of the time, it does almost nothing. But, they will try to fix it up as good as new.

> "Input from external sources is frequently garbled, misdirected, and misinterpreted."

After working on it for eight weeks, they inform you that they've done all they can, explaining that a few of the glitches appear less severe, some but may be permanent and the load of lost data might never be recovered.

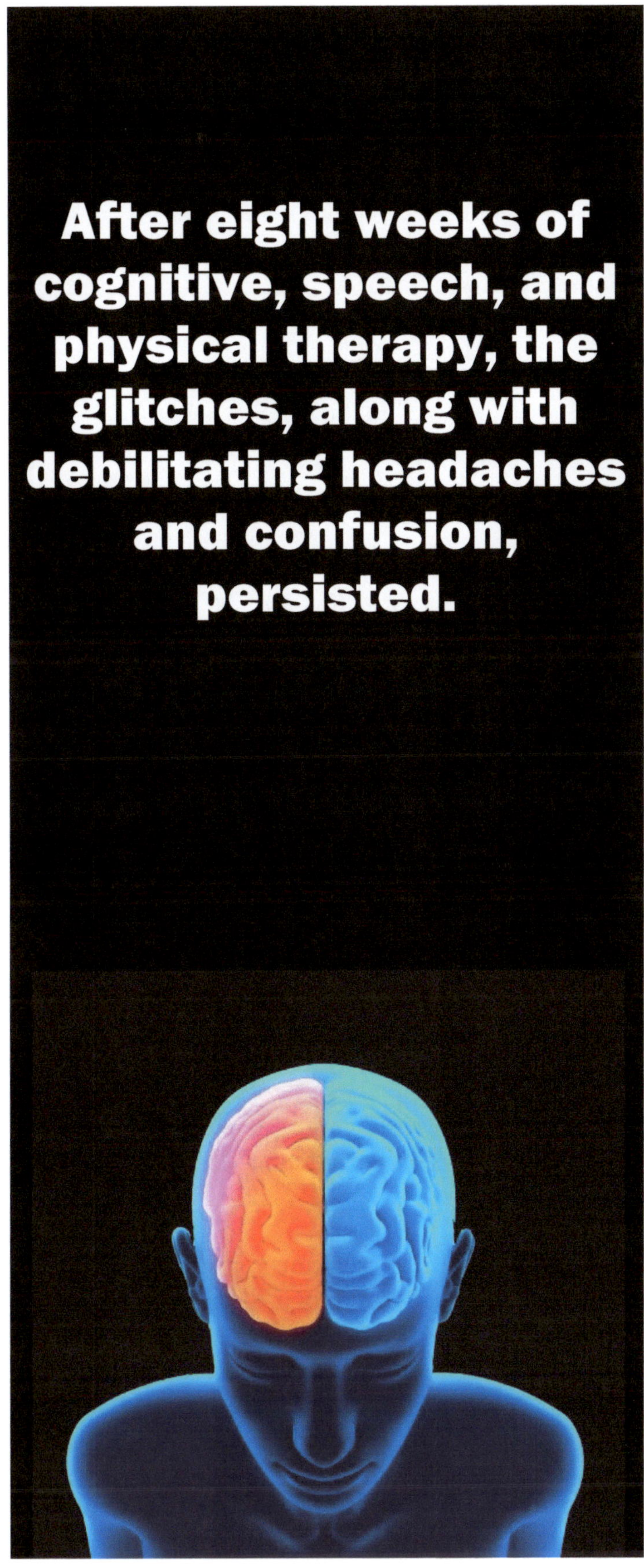

Which option would you choose?

    A. Toss it, and buy a new computer
    B. Keep using the old one, and get used to the glitches
    C. Keep using the old one, and try a "DIY" repair to reduce glitches

Did you choose A? Likely and logical, especially if you use it a lot.

Did you choose B? Not likely or logical, as it defeats the purpose of a computer.

Did you choose C? Highly doubtful, since the experts couldn't repair it and most people don't know a motherboard from an ironing board. For me it was, and remains, the only option.

The computer described above is my brain following an automobile accident that left me with a "mild" traumatic brain injury. After eight weeks of cognitive, speech, and physical therapy, the glitches, along with debilitating headaches and confusion, persisted.

Despite my limited understanding of the brain, much less the damaged brain, some inner part of me was pretty sure that just giving up, giving in, and accepting the finality of having *achieved maximum anticipated recovery* as stated on my paperwork, was simply unacceptable.

So, I didn't just choose option C, I embraced it. I still do hours of therapy every single day. I still have glitches. It's been six years.

Notice I said "mild" TBI. That is the diagnosis that the medical community uses to label this widely varying and often disabling condition. It's one that I view as anything but mild.

Like a malfunctioning computer, people with TBI tend to look fine on the outside, often with few physical tell-tale signs, and we try to limit circumstances or avoid situations that would make deficits more apparent.

Worse, we can't really explain the little horrors we experience several times a day, or the debilitating ones that occur several times a month. When we try, it's an exercise in futility, frustration, and most often results in a crushingly lonely sadness.

Whether a computer or a brain, it's clear that these glitches aren't mild. While TBI in general isn't readily understood by the majority of people to begin with, an adjective like "mild" only serves to exacerbate the effects of the condition with the misconceptions and misplaced expectations it creates. Family, friends and total strangers hear the word mild and can't see the injury, so some feel free to comment, question, or give their opinion. "Why can't you work?" "Why can't you drive?" "Wow! That was an inappropriate thing to say." "I think you're faking." "This TBI thing is an excuse to shirk your responsibilities." "Why are you crying?" "Everybody forgets sometimes." "You are still you." "You're lucky, it could have really been worse." "You look fine to me." "If you'd just try harder." What's more, a computer cannot feel physical pain or emotional anguish - additional gifts from the TBI Gods.

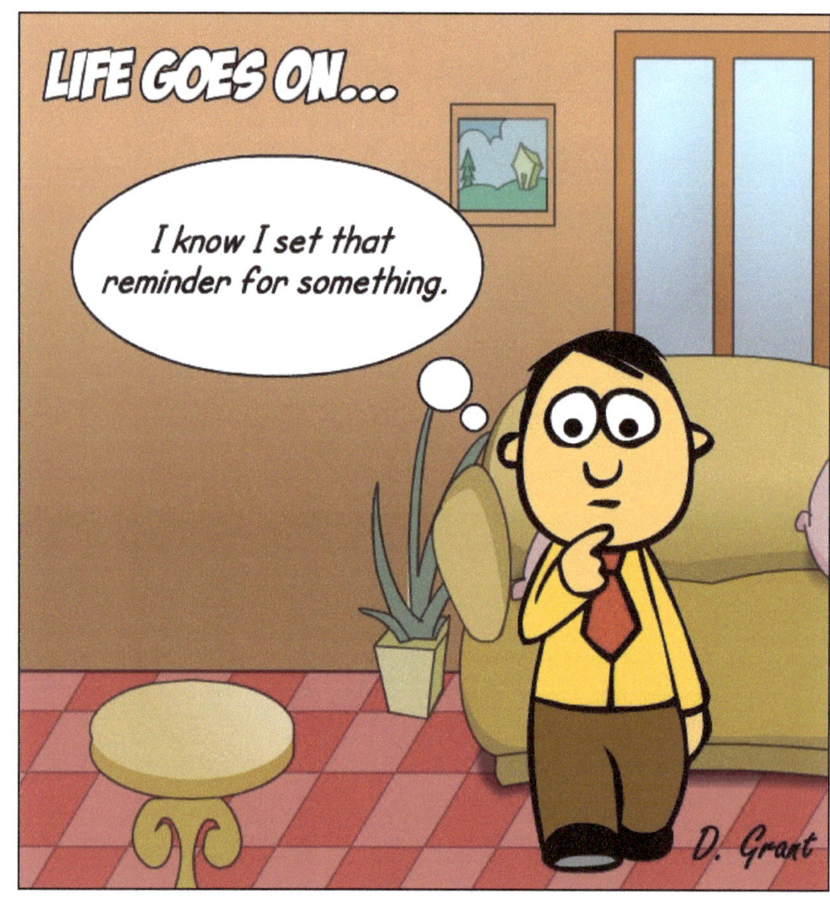

My point is that, sticks and stones aside, the word "mild" has the real-world consequences of further hurting survivors of brain injuries in ways the medical community has either not considered, or is choosing to ignore.

In part, it is a matter of conditioned perception of the word based on the typical meaning and use of the adjective. Perception and reality are not always the same thing, but we think they are. People tend to react based on perception as if it is reality. For example, if you perceive that the bug flying toward you is a wasp, you're going to react as if it is a wasp, by avoiding or swatting at it, even if it's really just a beetle. A "good" liar is actually one that is perceived as being truthful. A person driving a new Jaguar is perceived as having money.

How is the adjective 'mild' perceived? Mild weather is pleasant. Mild spice isn't very hot. People rarely stay home with a mild cold. A mildly amusing joke isn't all that funny. Essentially mild denotes pleasant, no big deal, not having much of an effect, or certainly not something that would inhibit essential or routine functions. So, telling someone I have a mild TBI doesn't allude to the number or kinds of effects I experience, does it? (See the list of my personal glitches) No, it does not.

It's time to find another label for the challenges we live with. At least something that doesn't mean pleasant and having little effect. It's not just a misnomer, it's an insult that perpetuates faulty perceptions and a lack of understanding, empathy, and accommodation, coupled with unreasonable expectations and negative character judgments.

Believe me, I'm grateful for every modicum of progress I've made, but the daily challenge of performing simple tasks, formulating a thought or an utterance, or recognizing the painfully apparent misconceptions someone has about what I'm going through makes the added slap of a term like mild, with all its gentle ramifications, an insult to injury. It makes the difficult and ongoing journey even harder.

It's one of the few things about this unasked-for horror that could easily be remedied. These are just some of the MILD TBI glitches that I am still working on through frustration, anger, fear, tears, hope, and utter stubbornness to reduce, circumnavigate, or learn to accept and accommodate. Feel free to cross off the ones you consider to be MILD.

- I get vertigo and fall over for no reason
- I can't drive for too many reasons to explain
- I can't go in stores because of the lights and noise
- I often can't eat because I'm nauseated so often, or I don't eat, because I forget to
- Sometimes I have no idea what I am doing from one minute to the next
- I can't cook when I'm alone because I forget I'm cooking (I've had a couple close calls with fire)
- I have long-lasting horrible headaches several times a week
- I can't ride in a car without getting sick and panic attacks (Limbic system)
- I can't remember if I've taken my meds or not
- I can't control my body temperature - freezing, hot and sweating
- I can't swallow completely and choke frequently, always congested
- I often can't recall words, or when I can, I can't formulate them with my mouth
- Sometimes my legs still don't respond properly to the walk command-jerky gait!
- I misunderstand what others say, or the intentions of what they've said
- I can't tell when people are joking, or I think they are, when they're not
- Sometimes there are no words at all, or the wrong one comes out - surprise!
- I smell noxious odors that aren't there and smell things that are, long before anyone else
- I can't sleep at night or regulate my circadian rhythm
- Sometimes made-up nonsense words are all I have to communicate with

- I have super sensitive hearing, but suffer poor discrimination during conversation
- I can't do two things at once, like walk and talk
- I laugh or cry at inappropriate times and without reason - hate that
- My verbal filter is gone - I unintentionally blurt out whatever pops in my head
- I can NEVER satisfactorily explain what I'm really experiencing
- Despite a loving family, I am painfully isolated and feel no one understands
- I feel like the "real me" is in there somewhere, just wandering and lost in a not-so-fun house

Life after brain injury is not easy. Dealing with my day-to-day glitches as best I can has allowed me to move forward in my life, not in a way that I ever expected, but in a way that works for me.

Meet Ali Blaylock

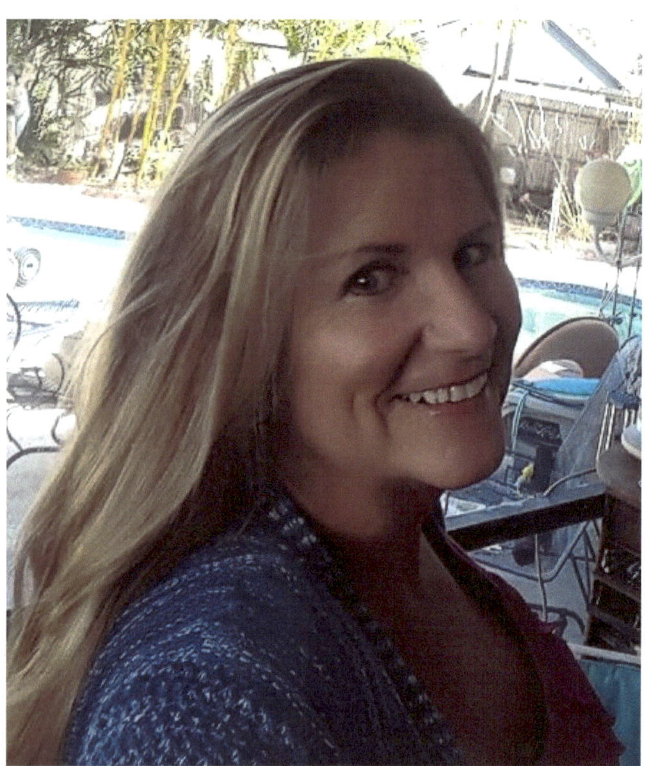

An author, artist, and certified sign language interpreter, Ali Blaylock is a six year TBI survivor as a result of an automobile accident that occurred when a driver illegally turned into her path.

She served as lead educational interpreter for the Palm Beach County school district, focusing on language acquisition and equal access, proposing best practices and innovative strategies that are still implemented today.

Since 2012, Ali has not been able to work, drive, travel more than short distances, and rarely ventures out of her home, but is not idle. She continues daily self-directed therapy aimed at improving cognition, speech, balance, and short-term memory, and hopes to publish her first fiction novel in the very near future.

Some of us think holding on makes us strong; but sometimes it is letting go.

-Hermann Hesse

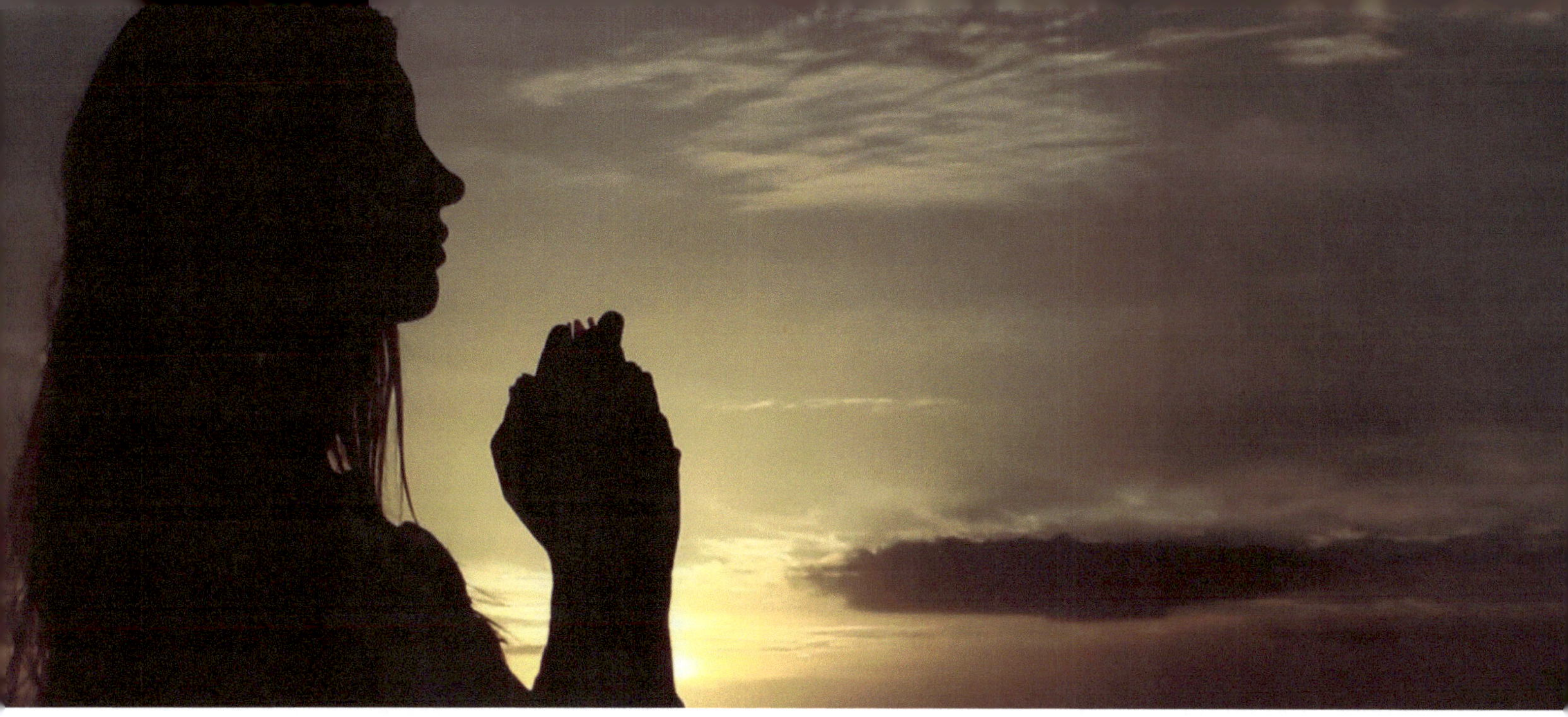

My Healing

By Debra Gorman

I could see the question in her eyes—and in the tilt of her head—and the wrinkle of her brow. I recognized the expression but her question was a silent one. Our chat had led us to this point: *Why doesn't your faith heal you?*

I wish she would come out with it. I would like to tell her that I will most definitely be healed, maybe not in this lifetime, but later. My faith tells me that the "inconvenience" of a brain injury was allowed by my Heavenly Father, not because he is a cruel ogre in the sky, but because he loves me too much to leave me as I was. There is something that I can give and something I can receive most effectively from this difficult experience. Oh, it has been difficult. I need a stronger word—arduous maybe? Formidable? There were times when I thought the weight of it would kill me.

> "There were times when I thought the weight of it would kill me."

But since it didn't, I decided to get down to the business of understanding it a little better, to submit to a higher power, one who could heal me if that was in my best interest. By this time in my life and experience, I desire what is in my best interest. I believe he allowed the brain injury in order to shape and mold me into someone better than I would otherwise be.

It's not that I don't still see doctors and hope for physical improvement, I do. It's just that my ultimate well-being does not depend upon improvement. I CHOOSE happiness. I CHOOSE to be content in my circumstances. My faith allows me to do that.

How? Why?

Because I have a long history with God.

Sometimes I examine the inner me and note the positive changes that have taken place since my brain injury. I am more patient, loving and understanding. I realize that God's love is bigger than I had thought. In the past, I was somewhat rigid in my beliefs. I thought I knew God, but I didn't, not really.

God gives me peace and grace as a result of trusting him. He is all knowing and all loving. My inability to understand everything that occurs in this world is my problem, not his—or hers. Actually, God doesn't need or have a gender.

I haven't always felt so hopeful. Six years ago, a few months after my brain hemorrhage, I hit a bottom. I remember having dinner at the kitchen table with my husband on a winter night. Outside, snow was falling and the wind was whipping it into big drifts. My dog sat curled up under my chair because that's where she was most likely to catch the food that fell from my fork as I tried to get it from my plate to my mouth. I am not naturally right-handed and have really struggled to learn to eat and write using my right hand. That evening, in the midst of dinner, my head fell onto my chest and I sobbed my despair.

My life has included many difficult blows, but never, EVER, had I felt more alone and sad than at that moment. I felt doomed. For a time I lost hope. How would I go on living? How could I bear to live as a… a handicapped person?

It was a night of anguish, but it was also a turning point. I did not want to live out my remaining time as a sad or bitter person.

It has been six years since my brain hemorrhage and subsequent subdural hematoma, but I have begun to be aware and truly grateful that my injuries were not worse. As it was, I narrowly escaped death. I have been given the gift of a future and time to do something worthwhile. I don't know if I have many more future days or few, I just want to use them wisely. I want to make a positive contribution in this world. I want to live open-hearted and open-handed. I want eyes that see possibilities instead of barriers.

I remind myself that God said his plan was to give me a future and a hope. That promise offers tremendous comfort.

Meet Debra Gorman

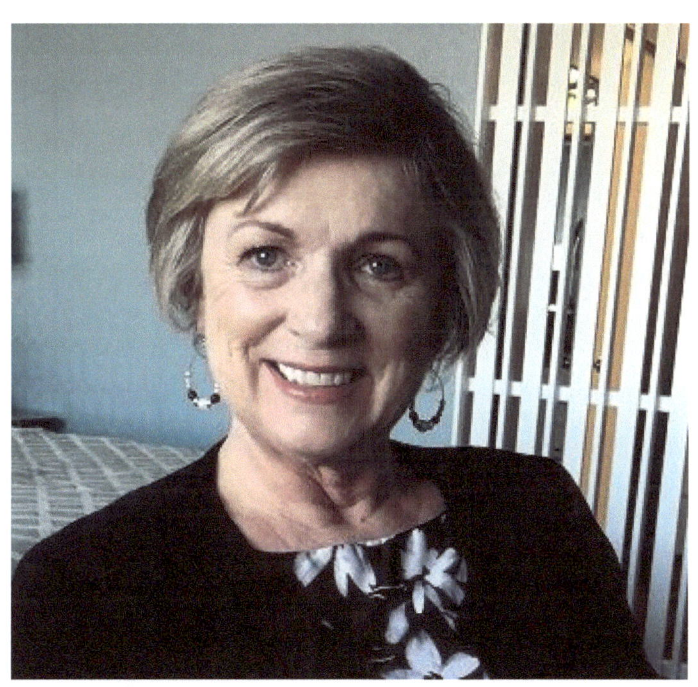

Debra Gorman was fifty-six years old when she experienced her brain injuries. The first was a cavernous angioma, causing her brain to bleed, and four months later, a subdural hematoma. She later learned that she also had suffered a stroke during one of those events.

At the time of the injuries, Debra was just becoming established in her new career as a Registered Nurse. She had been married only six years to her beloved. She had also been very active, hiking, backpacking, biking and weight training.

She finds a creative outlet in writing. She is able to use a keyboard, tapping keys with her non-dominant forefinger and thumb. She enjoys writing for her children and grandchildren and has written articles that have been published for hospice. Currently, she writes for her blog, entitled Graceful Journey and can be found at debralynn48.wordpress.com

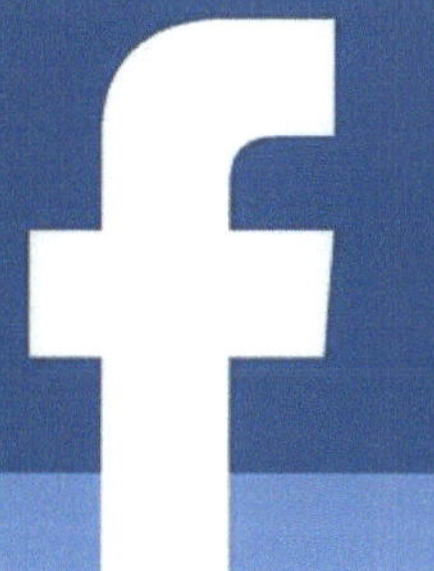

CONCUSSION

A concussion is a mild form of traumatic brain injury (TBI) caused by a bump, blow, or jolt to the head. Concussions can also occur from a fall or a blow to the body that causes the head to move rapidly back and forth. Doctors may describe these injuries as "mild" because concussions are usually not life-threatening. Even so, their effects can be serious. Understanding the signs and symptoms of a concussion can help you get better more quickly.

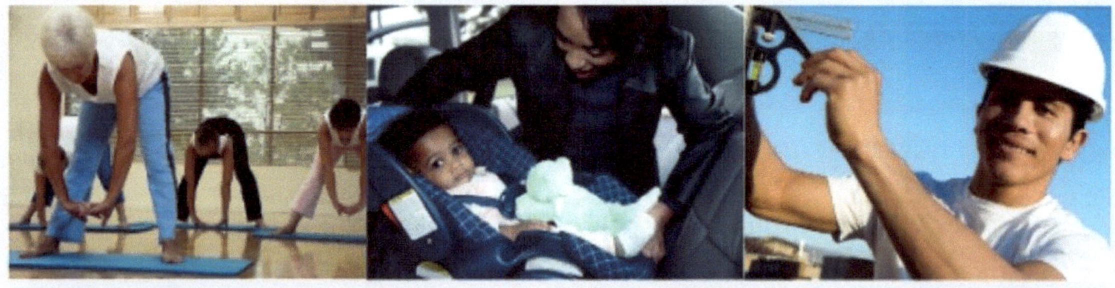

Leading causes of concussion

(seen in emergency departments):

- falls
- motor vehicle-related injury
- unintentionally being struck by or against an obstacle
- assaults
- playing sports

Graphic Credit: CDC.gov

Everything Has Changed
By Jim Martin

Since my brain injury, there have been times where I have felt vulnerable. For example, I recently attended a Super Bowl party at good friend's home. I arrived early as I had just adopted a new dog/puppy (Preston), and my hosts had a 10-year-old Golden Retriever, so was hoping to "find a friend" for Preston, which I did. The other guests arrived, the game began, and eventually I became unable to follow the conversation. Just prior to half time, I went home and enjoyed the game.

I realize that isolating is not helpful; yet I also know that I need to take care of myself. This can be a bit of a quandary in such a notorious social setting. That led me to consider the concept of vulnerability, something I seldom, if ever, considered prior to my brain injury. Now, it smacks me in the face. Vulnerability can mean several things to many different people.

Not wanting to think of myself as vulnerable, one of the first things which come to mind is weakness. Stated differently, I wanted to be useful, but I definitely did not want to be used, and that was not my perspective when offering assistance or even simply being social.

From a dictionary definition, vulnerability can mean being capable of, or susceptible to, being wounded or hurt, physically or emotionally, or being open to moral attack, criticism, or temptation. But, as I have learned over the past seven years, vulnerability can be having courage despite my impairments.

Vulnerability can include asking for help, saying no, standing up for myself, respectfully acknowledging that I'm afraid at times.

That leads me back to seeking balance in my life. I read an article a few years ago about balance in the context of riding a horse. It had a profound impact. In essence, there are many parallels. For example, the horse cannot carry my emotional baggage and still perform. Similarly, in spite of my invisible deficits, those around me cannot and should not need to suffer my deficits. So, balance becomes huge for me. Holding on to past hurts, accidents, grievances, worries and resentments affects no one but me. I'm becoming more and more comfortable which requires me to experience more vulnerability. I suspect many can identify when I say that everything has changed. But, with a healthier perspective, it's not too bad. I can now perceive life from my heart as compared to my head. It is a different, very different, life experience, but one that has permitted me to embrace all that life has to offer.

Meet Jim Martin

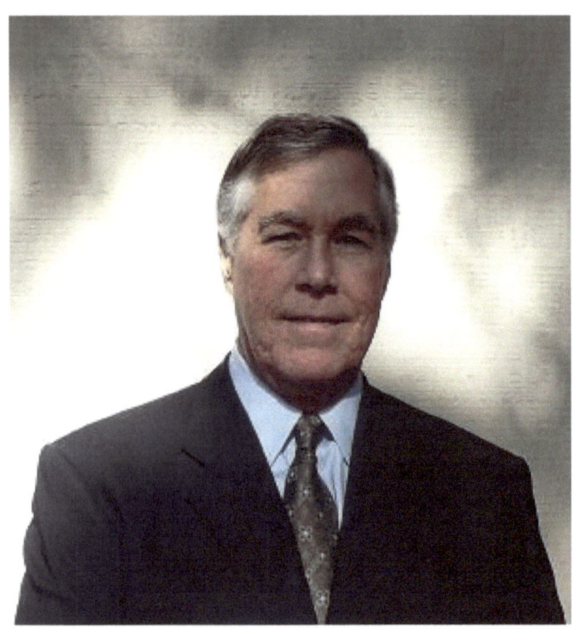

After 30 years practicing law as a trial attorney primarily representing physicians in medical malpractice litigation, Jim is a brain injury survivor whose career ended in December, 2010 when he experienced a significant traumatic brain injury, and resulting permanent memory impairment.

Following an extended period of time learning to accept his new reality, he now volunteers with the Alzheimer's Association, where he is a Board member, attends support group meetings with Brain Injury Connections NW, is a member of Brain Injury Alliance of Oregon, and volunteers at a local Portland, Oregon hospital.

To stay connected with the legal community, Jim mentors newly admitted lawyers with the Oregon State Bar.

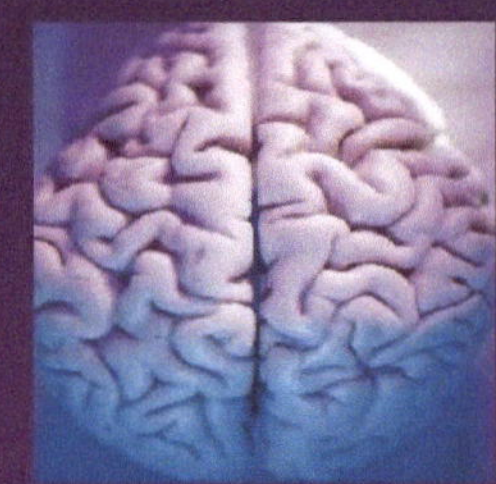

A bump, blow, or jolt to the head can cause a concussion, a type of traumatic brain injury (TBI). Concussions can also occur from a fall or a blow to the body that causes the head to move rapidly back and forth.

Some symptoms of a concussion are:

- Headaches that won't go away
- Having more trouble than usual remembering things or concentrating
- Confusion about recent events
- Feeling tired all of the time
- Feeling sad or anxious
- Becoming easily irritated or angry for little or no reason

Graphic Credit: CDC.gov

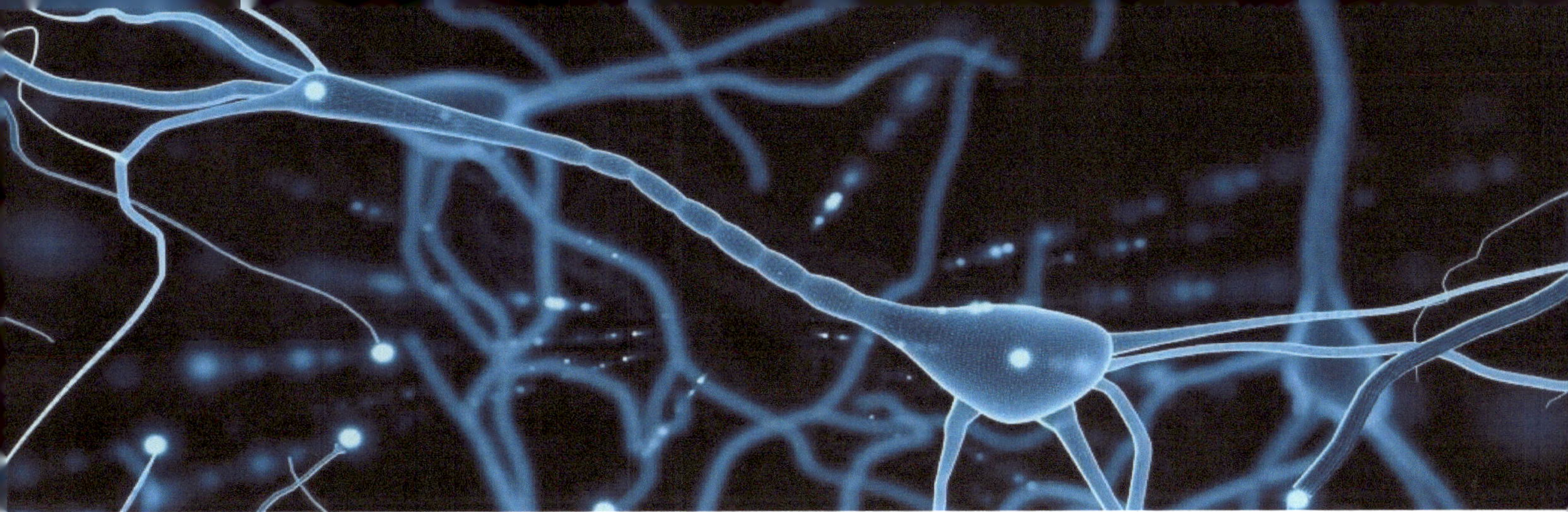

A Stroke of Faith

By Mark Moore

On May 11, 2007, I knew all about life! That's right! Things were good and I knew where I was going and what I was doing. I was pretty much in control and I liked it like that!

The next day, May 12, 2007, everything changed. Just twenty-four hours later, I was down for the count. I was no longer in control of anything. I was fighting for my life.

My stroke moved me a little closer to my life's purpose. In those first weeks of simply struggling to survive, I didn't have much sense of anything, much less a changed direction, or a new plan for my future. I just wanted to take one day at a time and understand whatever normal was going to be for me from then on.

As I continued on the path to recovery, after surviving two strokes and an operation to relieve the pressure around my brain, I knew how fragile I was. I understood how fragile life really is. I rested in a coma for nearly six weeks, giving my body a chance to try to renew itself and when my eyes were opened, I started seeing things in ways I had never seen them before. I was touched by a stroke of faith, and an amazing flow of family love and dedication, and the blessing of friends and caregivers.

I may have thought life was challenging when I was the CFO of start-up companies, but I did not know what challenging was. I had never experienced the pressure of trying to learn how to tie my shoes, or the embarrassment of not knowing how to write a check. After all, I was a CPA, a guy that knew how the world of money operated.

> "In those first weeks of simply struggling to survive, I didn't have much sense of anything, much less a changed direction."

God didn't want the "I'll see you on Sunday!" guy. He wanted the "I'll see you every day, guy!" He wanted me to realize that my spirit needed to be re-energized right along with my body. How did He do it? He did it through my caregivers, my family, and my friends. Together they managed to give me a stroke of faith that makes a difference in my life every day.

When I had finally gotten back on my feet, my friends were amazed that I didn't want to get right back into my old work life. They were awed that I didn't want to play basketball, a game I had loved ever since I was a kid in Jamaica, Queens. Slowly, I caught on to what the new game of life was all about. It was about surrender. That's right. It was about giving up everything that I thought was important and replacing it with the things that are truly important. It was about giving from the heart and not just from the resources I had available to me. It was about showing up for my wife and my children and my friends in ways that I had missed in my over-worked, exhaustive entrepreneurial life. It was about standing still.

As my body started working with me, helping me to walk again and think straight and letting me understand that I was okay, I started being drawn to my faith in new ways. I struggled to learn more of what He wanted. I wanted to understand what it would mean to leave my old life behind and pick up from this new point and move on.

It's funny, but I had spent a lifetime trying to be sure that I could be independent. I didn't want to ever rely on anyone else for the things I needed to provide for my family. I thought that getting ahead was about establishing myself in the world as a good man and an able provider. Now, it turns out that those desires were good things. They were good things, but they weren't enough and they weren't moving me closer to the goal.

As I learned to walk again, breath by breath and step by step, I also learned to walk a little closer to God.

I learned that independence was not the key. Learning to rely on others was not the key either. Learning to rely on God was everything. With surrender came acceptance of my new normal. With that acceptance came hope for my new life. I understood that I may yet have some physical limitations, but none of those physical issues could limit me from standing closer to God in my daily walk and offering Him all that I was then and all that I will yet be.

My family loved me back into better health and my friends gave me steadfast support so that I could keep making the effort needed to heal and embrace life. My caregivers were patient protectors of my mind and body.

If you wonder why you had a stroke or why you've had a brain injury, you may discover some medical answers. If you wonder why you are working hard to recover and regain a sense of normalcy, you may find answers in the faces of your family. But if you wonder why this happened to you, then I might suggest that your experience may well be the catalyst to a new you and a new life purpose. Surrender all that you were, accept all that you are and you will discover hope like you've never understood it before.

Meet Mark Moore

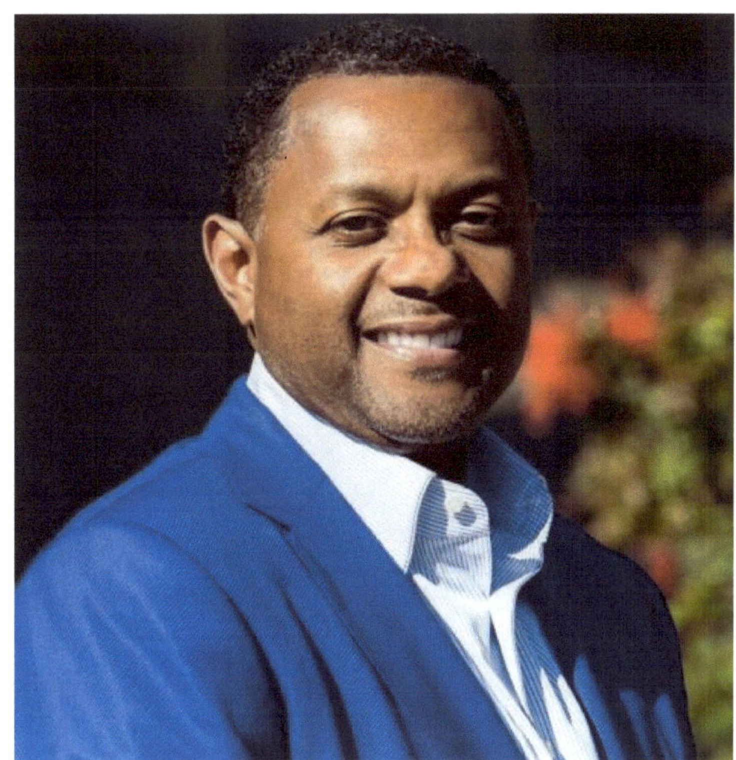

Mark Moore is a philanthropist and successful businessman. Along with his wife Brenda, a former nurse, Mark has established the Mark and Brenda Moore and Family Foundation, through which he supports advances in healthcare, education, culture and the arts, and Christian evangelism.

Prior to engaging full time in his philanthropic work, Mark was Chief Operating Officer and co-owner of Segovia, Inc., a leading provider of global internet protocol services to the US Defense Department.

Mark is also the Mid-Atlantic Ambassador for the American Stroke Association and the author of the memoir "A Stroke of Faith: A Stroke Survivor's Story of a Second Chance at Living a Life of Significance." More about Mark can be found at www.astrokeoffaith.com.

Finding Senior Housing can be complex, but it doesn't have to be.

Call A Place for Mom. Our Advisors are trusted, local experts who can help you understand your options. Since 2000, we've helped over one million families find senior living solutions that meet their unique needs.

"You can trust **A Place for Mom** to help you."

– Joan Lunden

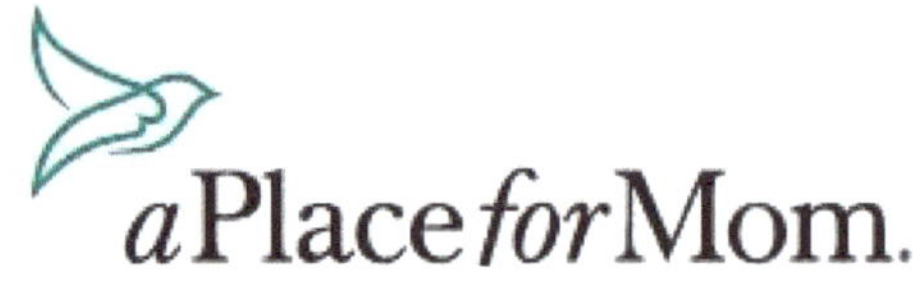

A Free Service for Families.
Call: (844) 578-9504

A Place for Mom is the nation's largest senior living referral information service.
We do not own, operate, endorse or recommend any senior living community.
We are paid by partner communities, so our services are completely free to families.

Tainted Within

By Seth Williams

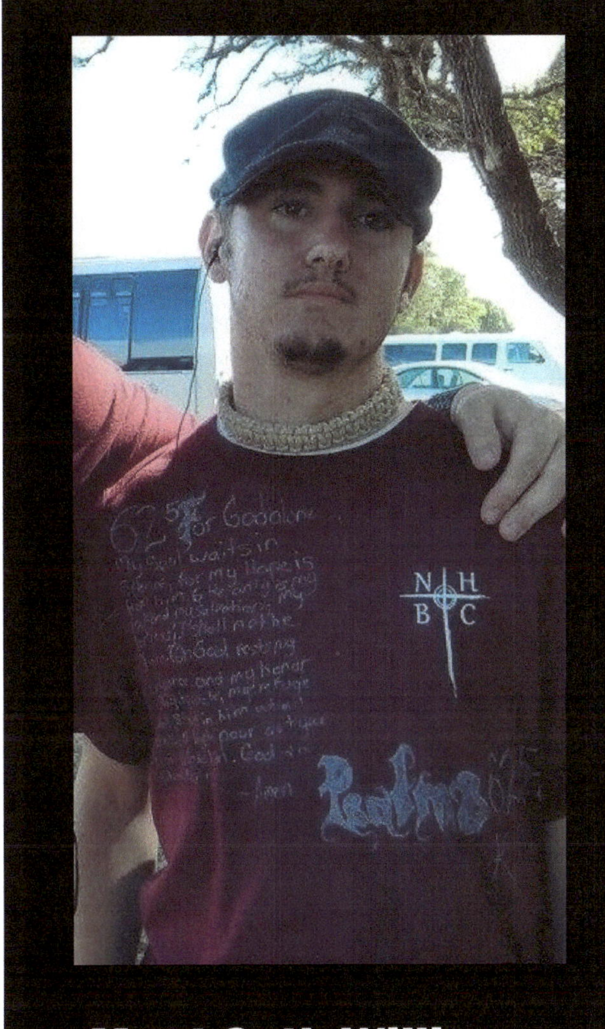

Meet Seth Williams

Seth writes…

"My name is Seth Williams. I am twenty-seven years old, and I am from Cary, NC. I had a Brain Tumor when I was nine years old. I had to have nine months of chemotherapy at that time. Chemo had many side effects and gave me scoliosis that I had to correct with surgery at age 18. My way of venting is writing poetry, and I like to draw the things I see. My idea of connecting with my peers is through my words I script."

When I was, young I had a debilitating encounter with a silent macabre

A disease that plagued my brain and stole a big part of my childhood

In the prime of my youth, I would collapse from the pain

Headaches and migraines were some of the symptoms I would get

I had an MRI to look at my brain; not sure what they would find

My Mom and Dad both received a call from the doctors at Duke

With news that would change my life and theirs forever

They had found a tumor hidden behind my cerebellum.

Surgery was scheduled for that next Wednesday. Oh, I was scared

My heart was beating like a drum on a drum line

Thoughts of my good friend Annah E. were roaming my head

As I inhaled the invisible gases of anesthesia, my mind had switched to standby

I woke up nine hours later with a bandage on the back of my head

Now to show for me brave feat all that remains is a scar

And a stitch in time could never compare to mine

A triumph to tell, but much harder to live

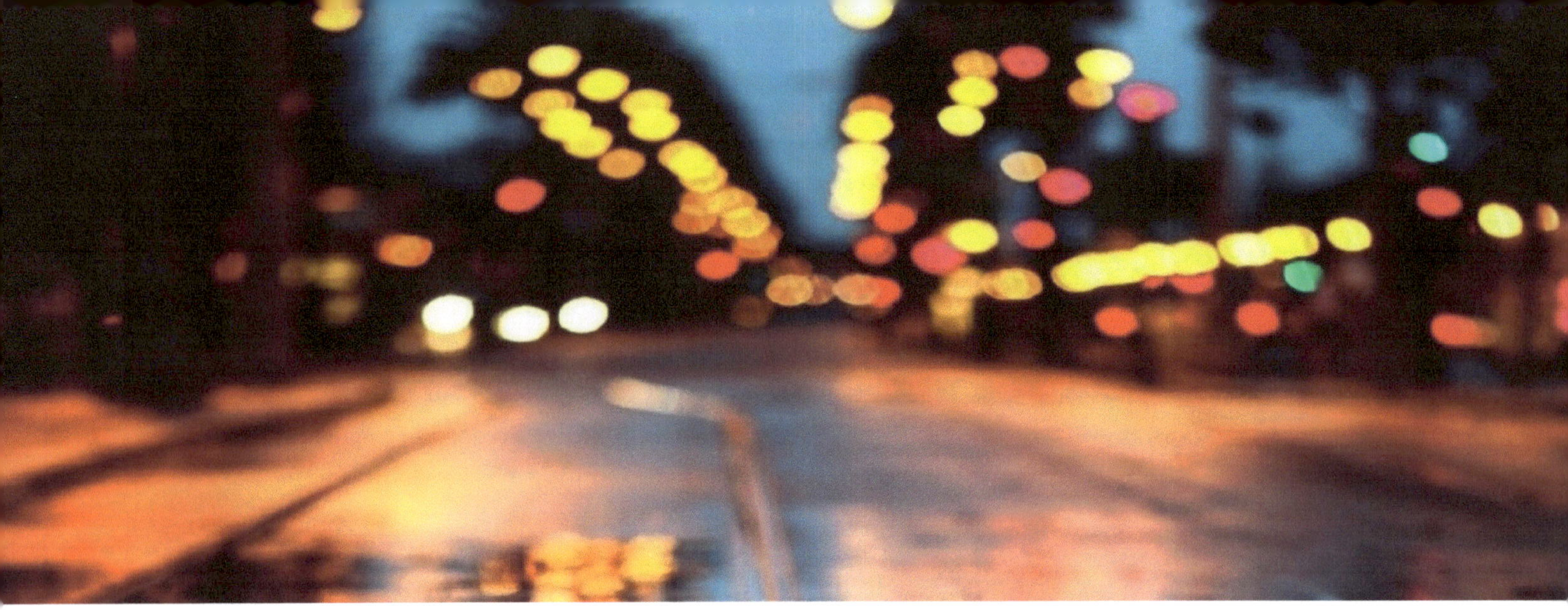

Trying to Slow Down
By Michelle Stokes

July 31, 2017, all seemed like a blur. I remember picking up my dog from the groomer with my two children in the golf cart. My dog was sitting on my lap as I drove away from the groomer's business and my children were buckled in the golf cart; however, I was not. Our dog jumped out of the golf cart and I remember looking back and seeing her tumble on the pavement but, that's it. I woke up in the Emergency Room by myself.

By some miracle the golf cart hit a speed limit sign and stopped, leaving the girls unharmed. I was in ICU for days and the recovery is still ongoing. I have been in speech therapy for months and resistant to being put on medication. There are multiple daily challenges. The largest challenge, and the one I have yet to conquer, is slowing down in our fast-paced society. Can it be done? I'm not sure.

"It took five months to adjust back to home life - caring for children, keeping up the house and being a wife."

It took five months to adjust back to home life - caring for children, keeping up the house and being a wife. The humorous, or not so humorous, thing about a brain injury is that as soon as one feels that he or she has conquered normalcy in life, he or she is thrown a curveball. Usually, it's a nasty curveball. I started a Master's program for Education. I was moving along quickly, doing well, and feeling like I could conquer the world. Next, I added in a part-time ESL job. Lastly, I started experiencing emotional meltdowns daily. I wasn't ready. It couldn't be done. I could not be a good mother, good wife, graduate student and teacher. It did not make sense. I was a: full-time English teacher before the accident, a good mom and a good wife. I was efficient. I was happy. I could multitask. I was me.

Now, I cannot hold a part-time job for two hours a day, be a graduate student and be a good mom and wife. The problem lies within me. I cannot say "no" to people. I added too many responsibilities too quickly. My first priority is to be a loving mother and wife. I want my family to feel loved. I remember being in the hospital room and thinking about never seeing my children again. I lost my sense of smell and will most likely never be able to smell them again, but I can hold them and give them all the love that I have.

It took five months post-accident for me to become an effective and loving mom. And it was hard. It was hard to get one child to preschool, one child to swim lessons, one child to gymnastics, put food on the table and remember all the things one needs to remember on a daily basis.

With the help of some compensation strategies, I have managed to return to being an efficient mother who needs much more help from others and many more brain breaks for herself. I cannot function without a daily agenda. Everything has a place; the keys go in a certain drawer, the backpack goes on a certain hook and so on.

Everything has a place. While there are days when I feel like everything is spinning out of control, I know that I can make it. It just takes time - time that society does not want to give. After learning from experience (always the hard way), I learned that one cannot jump back into the busy life. I thought a part-time job was manageable with grad school, but it turns out that it was not.

It took five months post-accident for me to become an effective and loving mom.

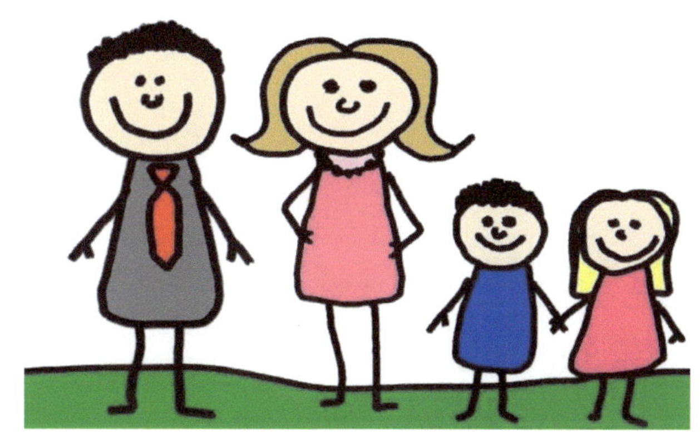

Now, I am trying to embrace a slower lifestyle. It is not easy, but it is worth it. I get to cuddle with my children. I have the opportunity to make them breakfast. No, I am not teaching other individual's children, but I am teaching my own children.

Through the horrible accident, I am teaching them compassion. I am teaching them to not be judgmental. Without experiencing the accident, I would have never slowed down. I would have kept running the rat race of the American lifestyle.

I am experiencing and seeing now all of the things I was unappreciative of before the accident. I did not take time to watch them smile, hear them laugh and experience the true blessing of life. I have taken the phrase "hurry up" out of my vocabulary. There really is no need to say "hurry up." It causes unnecessary anxiety and stress. I cannot "hurry up" the healing process and my children do not need to "hurry up" through life.

I like to think that TBI survivors are the rebels; the ones who tell world they will not embrace the fast-paced lifestyle. Life is too short to live at the fast-paced tempo and when one does live at that speed, it is horrifically dangerous. Be grateful for another day; a day where one can enjoy the simple things in life.

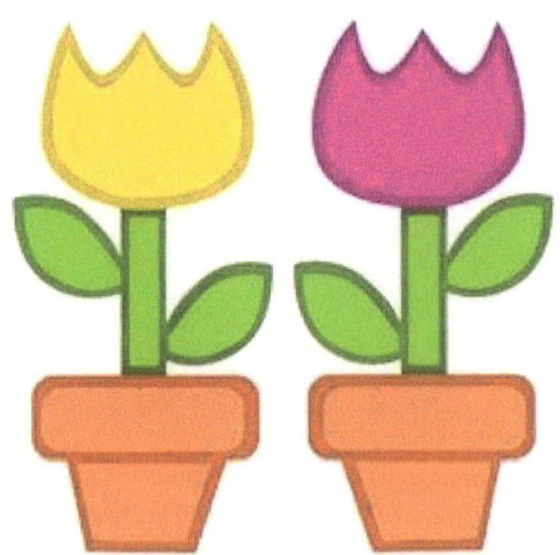

Meet Michelle Stokes

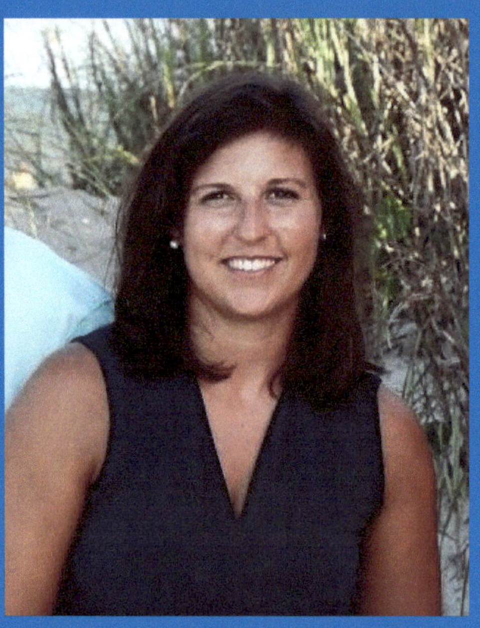

"My name is Michelle Stokes and I am 33 years old. I am a wife and a mother to two beautiful girls (ages 2 and 4) with a baby boy on the way. Prior to my accident, I was a high school English teacher for 10 years. I have always struggled with saying 'no,' which means my schedule has always been packed.

Though I am no longer pursuing my love for teaching through the means of a job, I have been given the beautiful opportunity to teach my children daily. I have learned that the accolades that come with living in a fast-paced society can be damaging to my home life. Every day I struggle with my recovery, but I always manage to find hope."

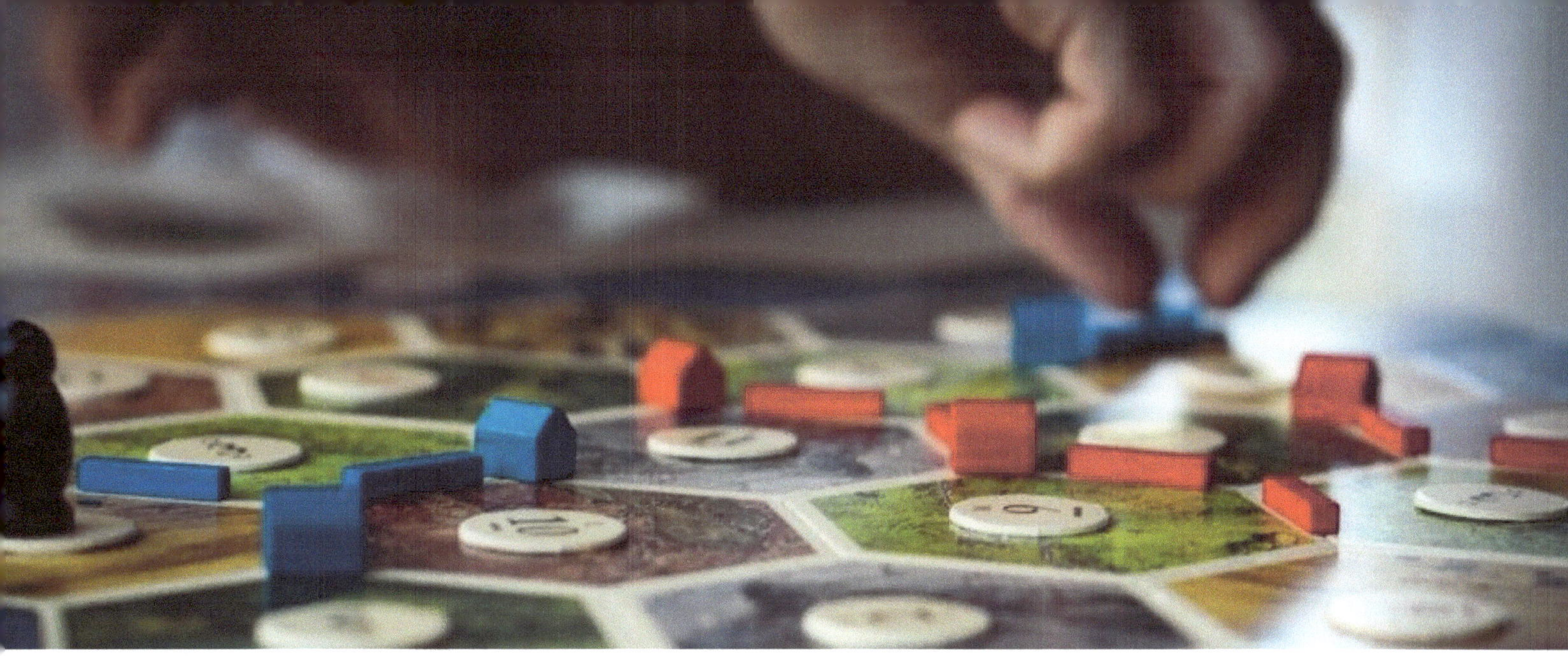

Fighting to Get Back
By Virginia Cote

My son, Rod, is an AVM survivor. It has been four years since his life was turned around, twisted about and thrown back at him. I find it helpful to read all the wonderful articles in the HOPE Magazine each month. They help me to understand what it is like for a TBI survivor, but only my son knows what it truly feels like for him each and every day. I think it is his depression that is hardest on me. He tries hard to keep it to himself as he fights to release the hold that it has over him. But I am his mother and I feel his hurts and frustrations.

I wish Rod could see what I see in him. Yes, he has had a brain injury and everything slows down for him. Words take longer to come out, while too much information coming at him all at once overloads his circuits and he has to shut down.

You can't spring things on him all of a sudden. He needs time to process information. But what I see in him is an incredibly smart man. I find myself going to him for advice all the time. Once Rod gets past the part where he thinks, "I cannot," "I do not know," "I am dumb," he gives me his good advice.

> "Too much information coming at him all at once overloads his circuits and he has to shut down."

When I ask Rod to help me with a project, his first reaction is, "I don't know how to do it." But if left alone he thinks it through and figures out how to start and once he starts it all comes back to him. Rod wants his brain to react immediately to everything but it won't. It has to process things first before it can respond. I am sure with more time he will learn to relax and have patience with himself.

As I read the articles in HOPE Magazine, I can see similarities in these TBI survivors: the loss of friends and even family members, because they cannot understand the new life these survivors must face; they look the same, why don't they think and act the same?

Too many people think recovery from a TBI is like on TV where they come out of a coma and are right back to their old selves. These are not bad people, they are just uneducated about brain injuries. It takes time, understanding, lots of praise and reassurance to help in their recoveries.

I also read how others like Rod get scared about things that look simple to us. Rod has trouble crossing roads. His eyesight was also damaged from the AVM. This and the brain injury highlight his fears - his very real fears. Because of his eyes and the slow reaction of his brain he cannot judge the speed of an oncoming car but this has not stopped him. Each crossing of a road is Rod meeting one more challenge head on.

When Rod is faced with a challenge, he keeps at it until he conquers it. I lost count of how many trips we made to Home Depot before he could actually buy something. Home Depot is still hard for him, but if we try to only find a few things at a time he does better. I can't express how proud I am of his determination to win over each of his battles.

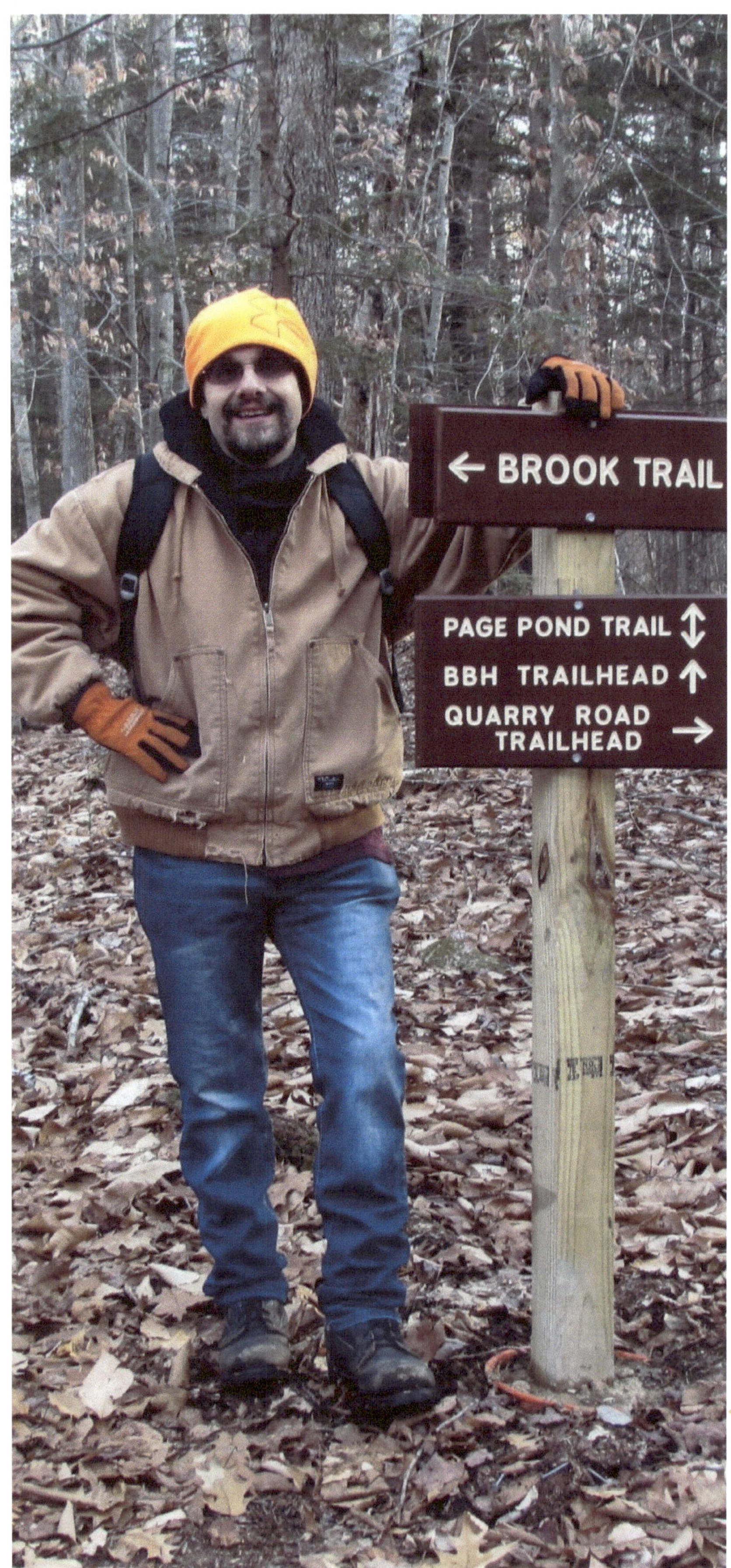

What I most admire about Rod is how he constantly hunts for things to do to challenge and improve his brain function. Reading is very hard and tiring for him. We have found a game to play that requires him to read questions off a card. He struggles but does not give up. Every night, Rod, his wife, and I play games for an hour or so. We vary which games we play. Some are more challenging for Rod so we let Rod set the pace as to how often to play them.

Only he knows what his brain can handle. We started by playing a dice game called ZONK. We now have seven games to choose from with UNO being our favorite. When we first started playing UNO, Rod had trouble with the colors. He couldn't remember the right names for each color so he started calling the color red, "tractor" after the new tractor he bought to mow our lawn. Then he called the color yellow, "Grampy" because that was my father's favorite color. Green became, "Gri Gri" (the name he used for his grandmother), her favorite color. Finally the color blue he calls, "blue" – go figure. Rod is the one that finds his own solutions on how to overcome his difficulties, proving he is smart.

> ## "Rod will not let his brain injury keep him from living a full life."

In the summer, Rod loves to walk in the woods. I will drop him off at a trail and pick him up hours later. He walks many miles and enjoys nature. He found out about Geocaching and that has been another exercise for his brain. Winter is the hardest time for Rod. It is hard for him to get outside. Cabin fever sets in and so does his depression. But today, there was no wind and the sun was out, so I dropped him and his wife Marlyn off downtown to walk around and get some needed exercise. Rod will not let his brain injury keep him from living a full life.

So, when I say I am incredibly proud of Rod it is mainly because of his determination to keep improving and fighting to get back as much as he possibly can.

Meet Virginia Cote

"I have been helping my son, Rod Stokes with his recovery from a brain injury. It has been a big learning process for me. He is the one that hunts and finds ways to challenge his brain. I support and encourage him and I am his transportation.

I have run a dog grooming and boarding kennel for over 50 years. In the past, I showed my dogs in Obedience Trials. The lessons I learned back then about patience, repetition, using small steps and lots of praise work for me today."

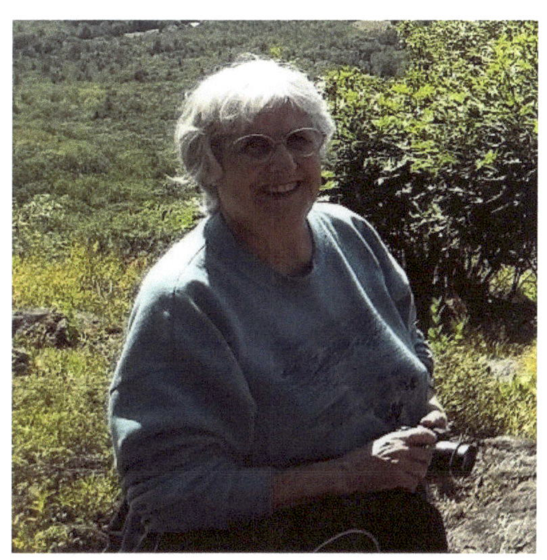

SYMPTOMS OF CONCUSSION

 **PERSONS OF ALL AGES**

"I just don't feel like myself."

Most people with a concussion have one or more of the symptoms listed below and recover fully within days, weeks or a few months. But for some people, symptoms of concussion can last even longer. Generally, if you feel that "something is not quite right," or if you are feeling "foggy," you should talk with your doctor.

Concussion symptoms are often grouped into four categories, including:

THINKING/ REMEMBERING	PHYSICAL	EMOTIONAL/ MOOD	SLEEP DISTURBANCE
• Difficulty thinking clearly • Feeling slowed down • Difficulty concentrating • Difficulty remembering new information	• Headache • Nausea or vomiting (early on) • Balance problems • Dizziness • Fuzzy or blurry vision • Feeling tired, having no energy • Sensitivity to noise or light	• Irritability • Sadness • More emotional • Nervousness or anxiety	• Sleeping more than usual • Sleeping less than usual • Trouble falling asleep

Graphic Credit: CDC.gov

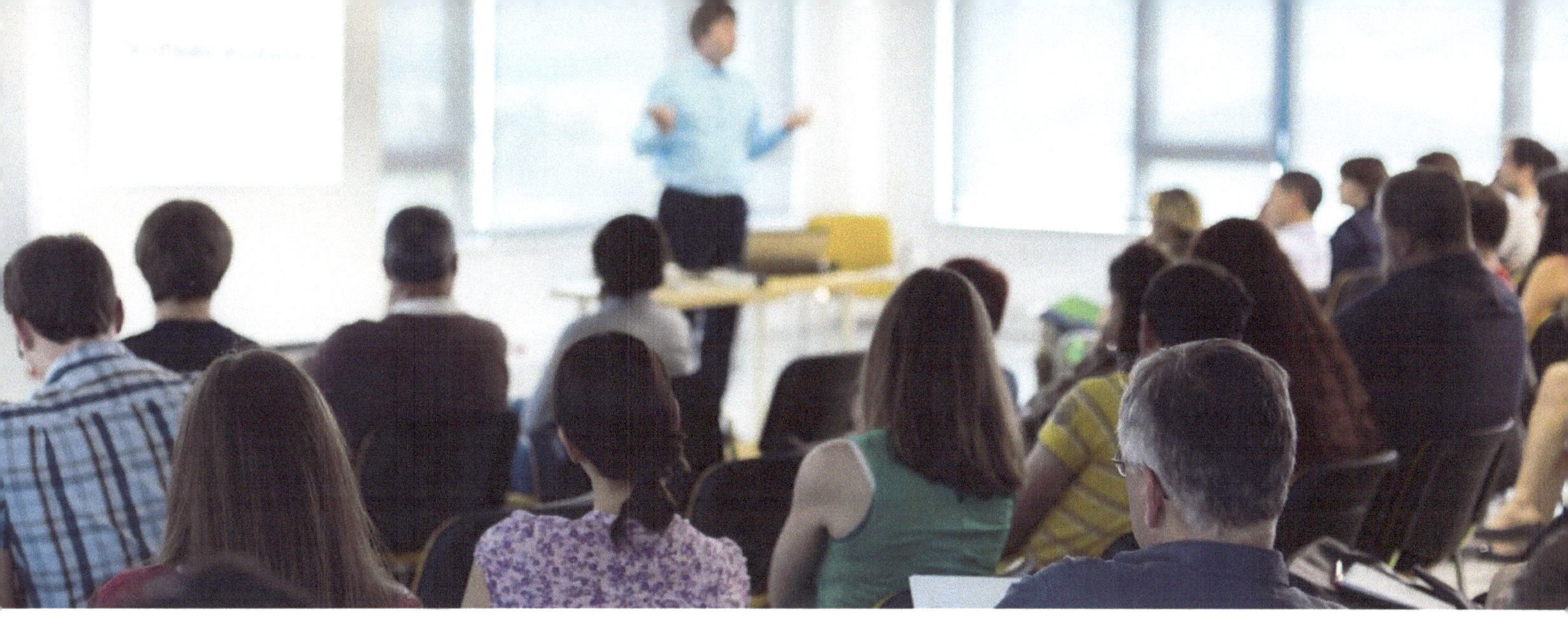

Educating Others
By Ted Stachulski

Every time I go to the Krempels Center in Portsmouth, New Hampshire, the members, staff, and interns inspire me. It is a community program for people with Acquired Brain Injury (Traumatic Brain Injury, Stroke, Brain Cancer, Anoxia from Heart Attack, etc.) There is so much love, caring and sharing of heartache that is always followed by words of wisdom and stories of courageous convictions and perseverance. Sometimes something special happens in a group that inspires me to write an article.

The goal of the Krempels Center is to reintegrate people with acquired brain injury back into the community. Members start by getting acquainted with the Krempels Community, which is housed in the Community Campus, a large three-level building with a full gymnasium, kitchen and dining area, and multiple classrooms. Then they're given opportunities to explore, participate in events, and provide brain injury education in the local, regional, nationwide and worldwide communities.

> "Brain Injury Survivors learn their quest to get back to being their old self again is like bailing out a sinking boat with a bottomless bucket."

Brain Injury Survivors learn their quest to get back to being their old self again is like bailing out a sinking boat with a bottomless bucket. Eventually, they learn (months, years, and decades later) their quest was not about trying to be their old self, but to embrace the new person they have become. This has got to be one of the hardest challenges after suffering a brain injury, which is often delayed by the survivor's own lack of education and misconceptions about brain injury, stigmas which prevent someone from asking for help and unwillingness to give up the life they once worked so hard to achieve and live.

At the same time, they must deal with people who don't understand what they're going through. Several members and I were given an ***Educating Others about Your Brain Injury*** worksheet in the Community Education group. Our group leader explained to us that outreaching to the greater community often starts with educating people we already have a relationship with, now or in the past.

Here is how I filled out my ***Educating others about your Brain Injury*** worksheet:

Who do I want to tell about my brain injury: Old and new friends.

Type of relationship: Friendship with classmates, teammates, Veterans, co-workers, neighbors, Brain Injury Survivors.

Why do I want to have this conversation: I miss and value our friendship.

Timing: Spontaneous and plan ahead.

How I'll introduce the topic: Via conversations and articles I've written about my Traumatic Brain Injuries.

Points I want to cover:

1. How was I injured?
From ages 5 through 17, I had many concussions, knockouts, and countless repetitive sub-concussive hits from playing sports. In 2001, I survived an accident that happened in the blink of an eye which could've killed me. Instead, it left me severely disabled.

2. Initial Diagnosis
A Traumatic Brain Injury (***TBI***) is a disruption in the normal function of the *brain* that can be caused by a bump, blow, or jolt to the *head*, or penetrating *head injury*. I was initially told by an Emergency Department doctor that I had a concussion and that I would be clear to go back

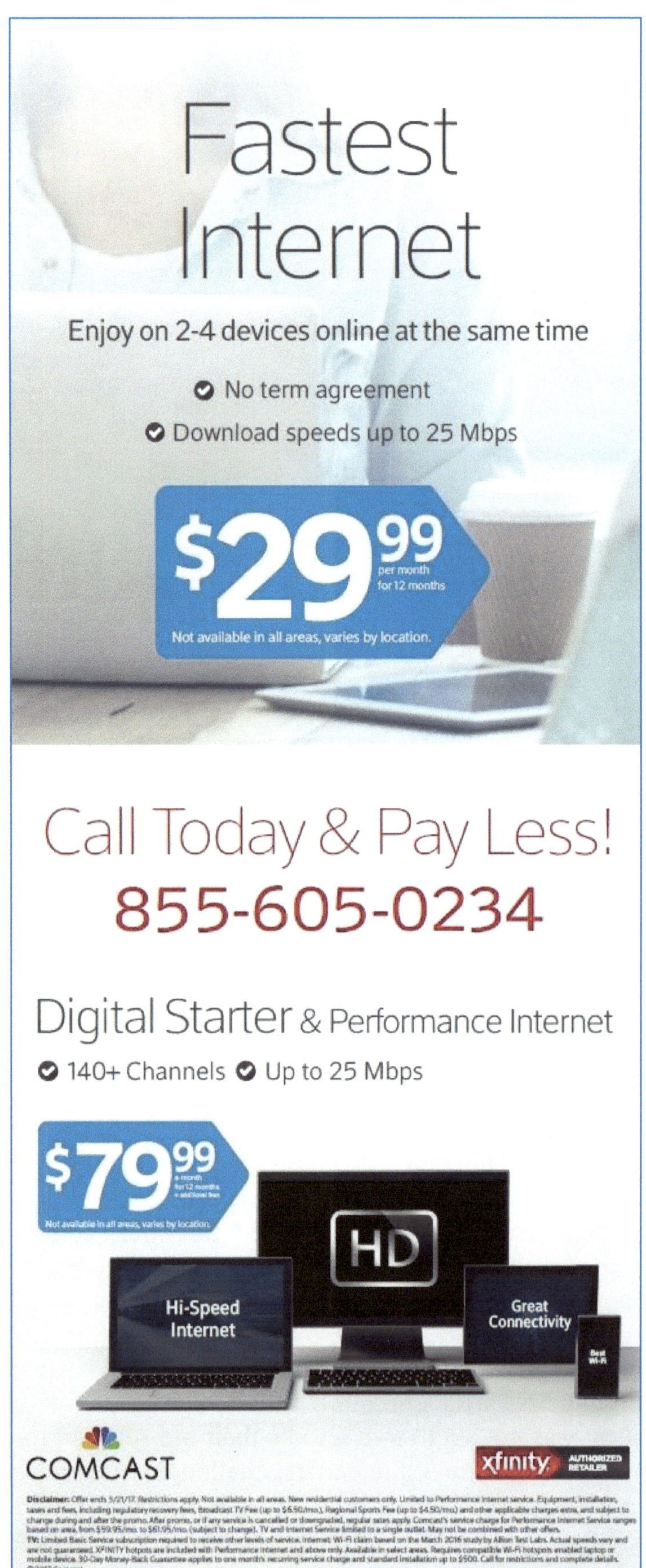

to work in three days instead of being sent to a rehabilitation hospital. With no rehabilitation, education or support my world fell apart quickly. Even though I look normal, I was badly injured. What looked abnormal at the time of my injury was immediately removed from my forehead or corrected with cosmetic surgery.

3. Bad Advice, Stigma, Denial and No Rehabilitation

While going through the motions of trying to live my life post-injury as I did pre-injury, I used bad and false information I had received from coaches, trainers and doctors about concussions and TBI as part of my recovery strategy. You may or may not know that I played in a high school football game with a concussion and got a second concussion which resulted in me dropping out of high school and almost taking my life. I think we all know how much misinformation has hurt so many athletes and Veterans and enabled them to re-enter games and battles while still suffering from a brain injury without ever getting the proper medical attention or given enough time for their brains to heal. I let stigma prevent me from asking for help when I needed it (Men don't ask for help! It's a sign of weakness!) Instead of reaching out for help, I persevered to keep my jobs and hobbies.

4. Employment and Hobbies

I lost 13 jobs in four years in complete fight or flight mode and had to stop all of my hobbies. I burned a lot of bridges and lost a lot of good friends trying anything I could to be the OLD ME.

5. Isolation and the Old Me

For several years, I was bailing nonstop and as quickly as I could, to keep the OLD ME afloat. Sensing I was losing the battle, I moved far away from my

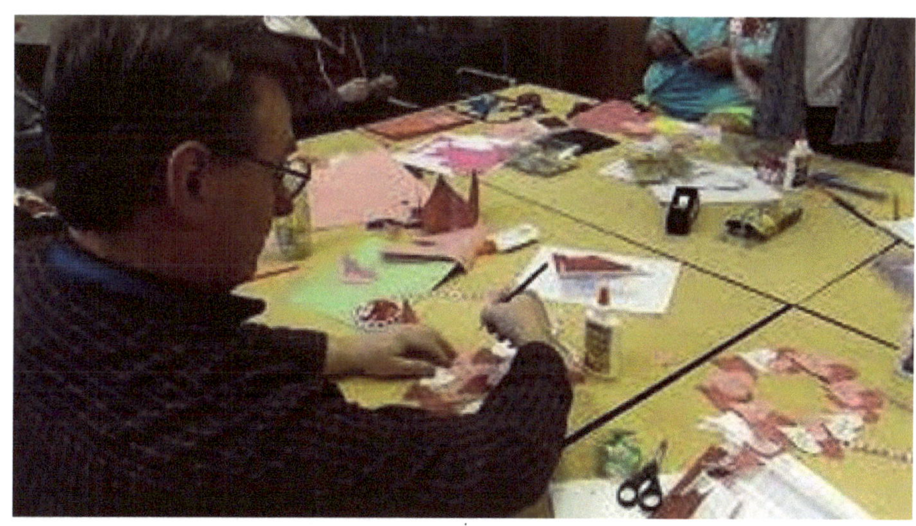

immediate family, friends and former co-workers to live in isolation because I didn't want anyone to see what was happening to me.

6. My Breaking Point and Diagnosis

In 2005, I went to the White River Junction VA Medical Center because I could not keep living in denial as my whole world fell apart. I was diagnosed with, and suffer from, Traumatic Brain Injury, Severe Post-Concussion Syndrome, and Post-Trauma Vision Syndrome. This means I have problems with attention, emotion, fatigue, processing delays, memory, vision, etc. I might also have Chronic Traumatic Encephalopathy (CTE), which is a neurodegenerative disease caused by a buildup of tau protein in the brain from all of those concussions, knockouts and sub-concussive hits you or others might have observed me get from ages 5 through 17. I don't let it bother me and will donate my brain to research when I'm done using it.

7. Uneasy Acceptance

It took a long time for me to accept that the OLD ME is not who I am today. My tipping point came after a Speech Therapist working for the Dept. of Veterans Affairs (who saw me struggle, break down and cry after trying to multitask) asked me, "What VALUE do you get out of doing this to yourself?"

8. Quality of Life

I have worked really hard to live the best quality of life I can and that's more important to me now than ever winning a championship in sports or getting a meritorious promotion in the Marine Corps. We owe it to our children and grandchildren to protect their brains and educate them about brain injury so they too can have a good Quality of Life.

9. Early Retirement

I've learned that even though I'm early retired, over the past 13 years I've worked hard to improve the quality of life for Athletes and Veterans with TBI and their family members. Instead of throwing blocks and making tackles in football, I break down barriers put up to prevent people with disabilities from getting the care they earned or paid for.

10. The Krempels Center

The Krempels Center helps me live a better life with brain injury. When I first became a member, I was very angry and tired of beating myself up every day with guilt and shame.

Other members taught me there is no shame in something I had no control over. I did not

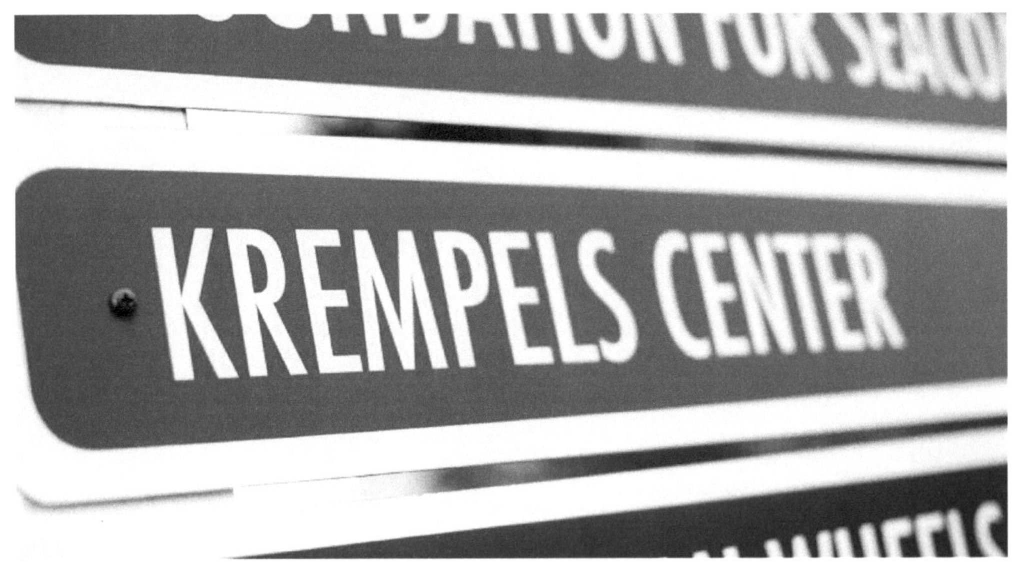

know all of those concussions, knockouts and sub-concussive hits would almost take my life as a teenager and then haunt me for the rest of my life.

I did not know I was going to be hit in the head by an 80-pound piece of steel in 2001. Three years later I'm not only surviving but thriving as a member of the Krempels Community, the brain injury community and in my local community.

My articles give a voice to Brain Injury Survivors who cannot advocate for themselves and educate those who want to know more about brain injury. There needs to be MORE of these facilities across the United States and abroad to help improve the quality of life for Acquired Brain Injury Survivors and their family members as well as train future Occupational Therapy, Speech-Language Therapy, Recreational Therapy, Social Work and Psychology Interns.

11. Friendship

A day has not gone by where I have not thought about friendships I had before and after my accident. The good times and the bad times, failures and triumphs and the memories we made and share in our hearts and minds. I'm not the same person you might have known in the past and I hope you have an easier time accepting it than I did. I MISS AND VALUE OUR FRIENDSHIP!

Meet Ted Stachulski

Ted Stachulski is a former multi-sport athlete, Marine Corps Veteran, Traumatic Brain Injury Survivor, creator of the Veterans Traumatic Brain Injury Survivor Guide, Veterans Outreach Specialist and an advocate for brain injury survivors, their family members and caregivers. Ted is a member of the Krempels Center, a nonprofit organization located in Portsmouth, New Hampshire, dedicated to improving the lives of people living with brain injury from trauma, tumor or stroke.

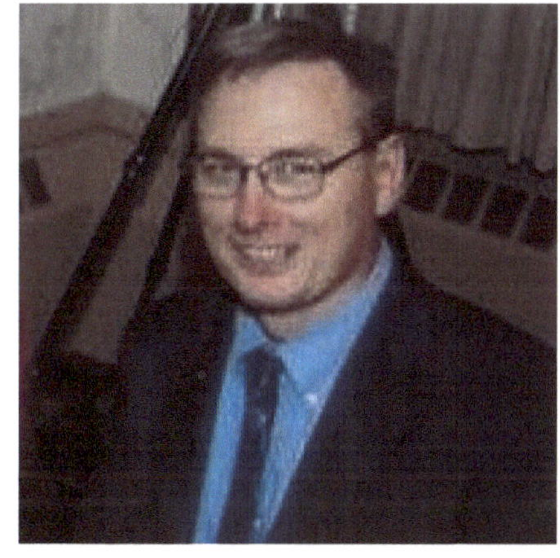

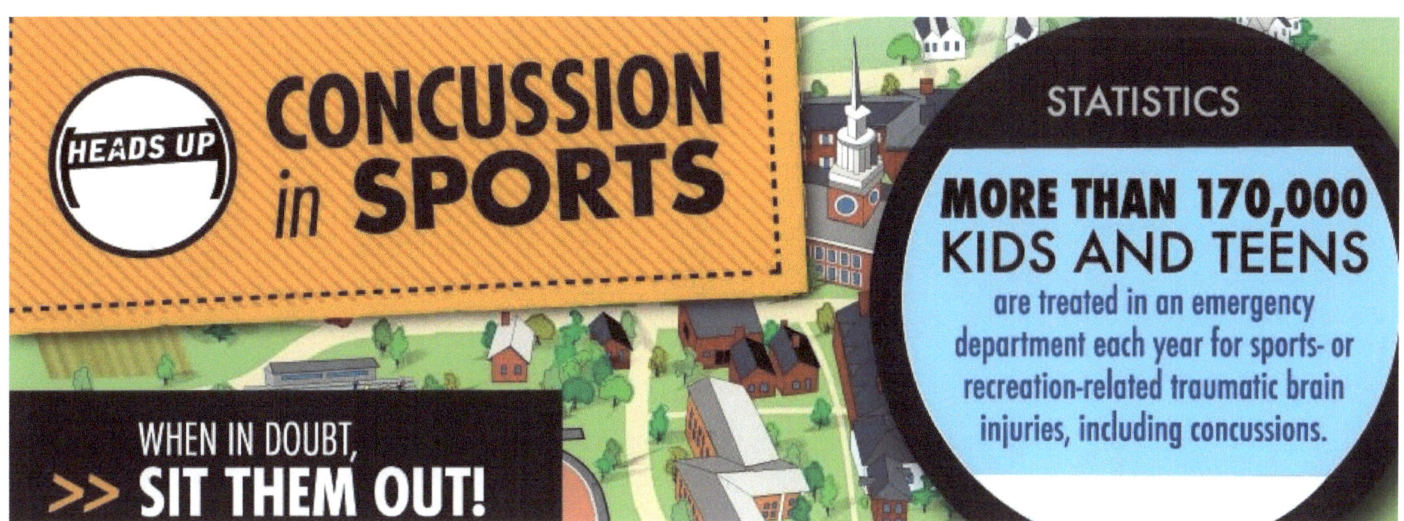

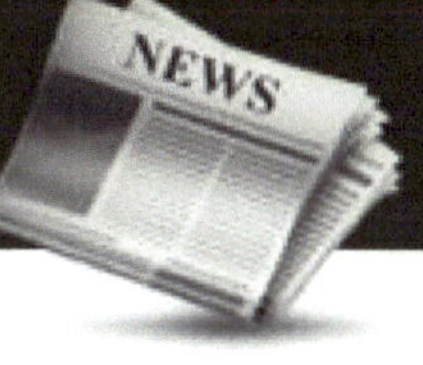

HOPE Magazine is very much a community effort. Sure, my wife Sarah and I compile all the content into an easy-to-read monthly publication, but it is the stories, and not their compilation, that our readership has come to appreciate.

Never have I heard a reader comment about a particular font that I have chosen. Feedback is always about the stories.

Recently, a reader let me know that he felt that our publication was too "religious." As I do whenever someone shares their opinion, I wondered if 1) there is merit to the comment and 2) based on the reader input, is there something we can do to better our publication.

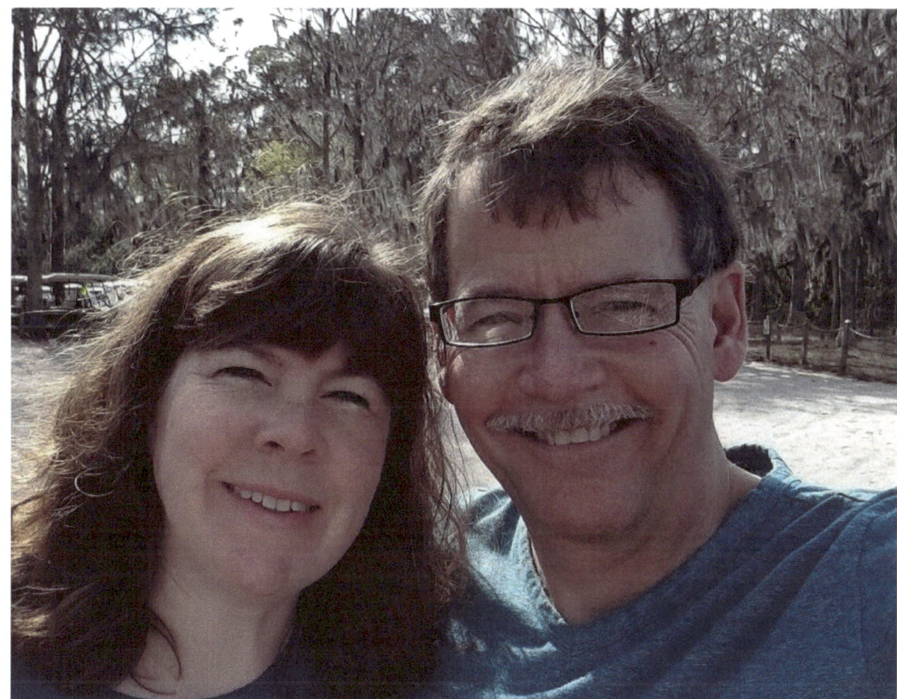

This month's issue has a few stories that talk specifically about spiritual experiences. Some speak of God, while others reference a Higher Power. Over the last several years, we have had submissions by contributors of many faiths. In fact, for many within the survivor community, there has been a strengthening of faith after brain injury. Perhaps it is because many of us, including myself, have faced almost certain death, only to come through to the other side, forever changed, but still alive.

We offer a platform for people of all faiths, or those with no faith at all, to share their experiences and hopes with others in the brain injury community.

~David & Sarah